A DOCTOR'S WISDOM FOR DIABETICS

The Sayings of Elliott Proctor Joslin

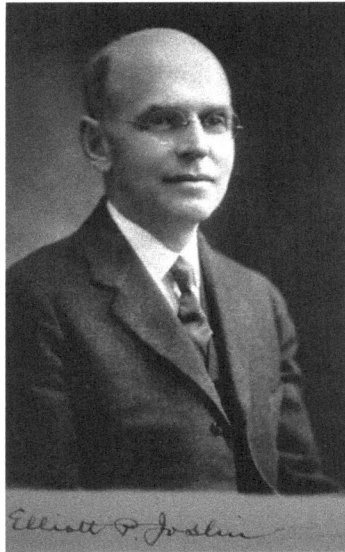

Elliott P. Joslin

S K Sinha

A Doctor's Wisdom for Diabetics

S K Sinha

ISBN: 978-0-6489470-9-7 (paperback)
ISBN: 978-0-6489470-8-0 (eBook)

Cover Design: Rockport, Maine. Lee Sinha

For all whose lives have been touched by diabetes

Also by this author

Joslin A Pioneer in Diabetes Care

The dawn of Joslin's career.

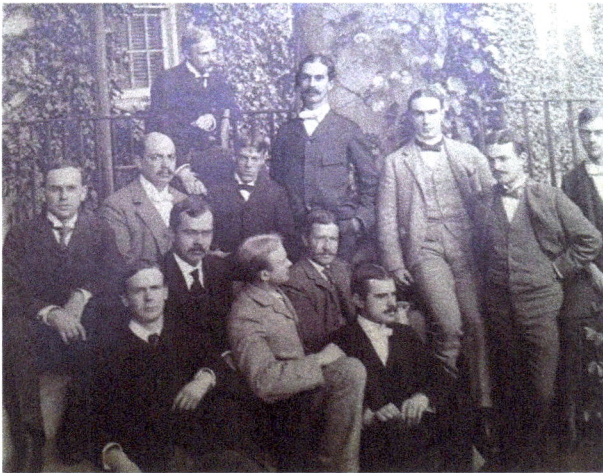

House officers at Massachusetts General Hospital 1897–1898.
Joslin is seated far left in the back row.

Introduction

"Joslin was best known for his inauguration of education for the diabetic patient."

DM Barnett 1998

Diabetes has afflicted mankind for thousands of years and continues to defy all attempts to control its rise let alone its eradication. Today most, if not all, developed countries face an increasing number of diabetics in their populations. With the condition now being seen to be on the rise in the less developed nations as well, diabetes can indeed be considered a pandemic.

Dr Elliott Proctor Joslin (1869–1962), regarded by many as the greatest diabetologist of the twentieth century, was born in Oxford, a small town in Massachusetts where his father owned a shoe-manufacturing business. Joslin, a Harvard professor and physician devoted his entire life to the study of diabetes and to providing care for those with the condition. He started medical practice in Boston in 1898, more than twenty years before the discovery of insulin in 1921, and worked to the last day of his life. Joslin died on 29 January 1962 at the age of 92 years. His practice remains the centrepiece of the eponymous institution in Boston and every year cares for literally thousands of men, women and children with diabetes. An outstanding scholar, the multilingual New Englander had burst onto the medical scene in 1916 when he published the first English-language textbook, *The Treatment of Diabetes Mellitus.* His opinions and observations on diabetes were based on the treatment of more than 52,000 diabetic patients seen in his practice. Joslin's innovative instruction manual for diabetics, *A Diabetic Manual for the Mutual Use of Doctor and Patient*, was published in 1918. With its rapid acceptance and popularity it easily outsold the textbook. Joslin wrote a manual to follow each edition of the textbook over the next 40 years, the last issue appearing in 1959 when he was 90 years old. A student of the classics, Joslin was fond of quoting from English, German and French literature as well as from books on medical history.

Most of these epigrams, aphorisms, quotes and personal stories are to be found in the manuals, because in these Joslin spoke much more freely – as much from the heart as from his mind – than he did in the textbook. He was not afraid to express personal opinions and could, at times, sound didactic. However, he always provided scientific reasons and appropriate references for his views by producing information from patients in his own practice or from scientific literature with which he kept abreast throughout his life. Indeed, he often corresponded with research workers based on information gained during medical conferences, even before the research paper was published, as he did at the time of the discovery of insulin.

Throughout his life Joslin strove to balance the demands of work ,with his studies and writings. The quote opposite, ascribed to Isidore, archbishop of Seville (c. 570–636), is felt by many to be his favourite. It appears on the flyleaf of his last two manuals and is also inscribed near the entrance to the Joslin Diabetes Foundation building.

Learn as if you were to live forever

Live as if you were to die tomorrow.

The Joslin instruction manuals were liberally sprinkled with biblical quotes.

Train up a child in the way he should go, and when he is old he will not depart from it.

Proverbs 22:6

James Baxter (1831–1921)

Baxter, a prominent merchant and scholar, was the husband of one of Joslin's maternal aunts. A powerful and vociferous supporter of the antivivisectionist movement, Baxter was opposed by Joslin largely because animal experiments had led to the discovery of insulin.

The verse opposite, a translation of a Persian poem by Baxter, was used by Joslin as an epigram.

*One who learns and learns
But does not what he knows
Is one who plows and plows
But never sows.*

Before the discovery of insulin, treatment of diabetes was restricted to dietary measures. There was little emphasis on educating patients at that time, but following the discovery of insulin in 1921 the dramatic effects of the hormone on diabetics convinced Joslin that instructions were essential. The supply of insulin for diabetics in America was not generally available till 1924.

Education of the diabetic was the experiment attempted in the first edition of the manual (published in 1918), but today it is recognised as a necessity.

(Preface to the third edition of Joslin's manual,1924.)

A lifelong interest in medical history had familiarised Joslin with medical pioneers like Louis Pasteur, the French microbiologist who had discovered that germs were responsible for souring alcohol which could be saved by heating, a process called *pasteurisation* after its discoverer.

"dans les champs de l'observation le hasard ne favorise que les esprits prepares."

Pasteur

Chance helps only the mind that is prepared.

Of the three most important rules for controlling diabetes, namely diet, insulin and exercise, Joslin considered exercise to be the most important.

Better to see how far you have walked than how much you have eaten.

Joslin's mother

Joslin was the son of Sarah Proctor, the second wife of Joslin's father, Allen Lafayette Joslin. She was the daughter of Abel Proctor, a wealthy leather merchant from Peabody. The strongly puritanical churchgoing mother was a major influence on Joslin throughout his life.

Sarah Proctor Joslin was a diabetic. She had lived with her son in the city of Boston after his graduation from Harvard Medical School. He had been his mother's physician to the end of her life and never forgot her strict adherence to the prescribed restricted diet.

Through much of his life Joslin had kept the identity of his mother from the readers of the manuals and his textbook, simply referring to her as "Case number 8". It was only in the last edition of his manual, issued in 1959 when he was 90, that he stated: "She was my Case No.8. ....Think of the effect of that one life upon the 52,000 cases which have come under my observation during 60 years of practice."

The quote opposite is from a poem by Ralph Waldo Emerson. Emerson was related to Joslin on his mother's side.

"Nor knowest thou what argument
Thy life to thy neighbour's creed has lent."
Emerson, "Each and All"

It was after Joslin's death, when some of his belongings were being cleared from his home, that a large framed photograph of the Methodist preacher John Wesley was discovered. Perhaps the zeal with which Joslin treated his patients with diabetes, and about which he was sometimes teased by his contemporaries, may have been the result of his admiration for Wesley who was also known for his enthusiastic evangelism.

Joslin worshipped at the Old South Church in Boston all his life.

Do all the good you can,
By all the means you can,
In all the ways you can,
In all the places you can,
At all the times you can,
To all the people you can,
As long as ever you can.

John Wesley's Rule
(From Elliott P Joslin, MD: *A Centennial Portrait by Donald M Barnett*.)

Following graduation from medical school, Joslin, like many medical graduates of his time, went to visit prominent medical universities and hospitals in Europe, particularly in Germany. It was here that he met and was deeply influenced by a professor in Strasbourg called Bernhard Naunyn, who impressed on the young medical graduate the importance of strict control of blood glucose levels, even in mild diabetes.

Strict control (of diabetes) pays.

A strong work ethic was very much part of the New England neo-Puritan way of life. Joslin pursued his goals academically and professionally with a single-mindedness verging on evangelical fervour.

Work shortens the day, but lengthens the life.

Feted throughout the English-speaking world, especially by medical colleagues, nowhere was Joslin respected more than in his home town of Oxford.

The stone mortar atop the baptismal font in the Oxford Congregational Church was a treasured indigenous relic held by the Joslin family for several generations.

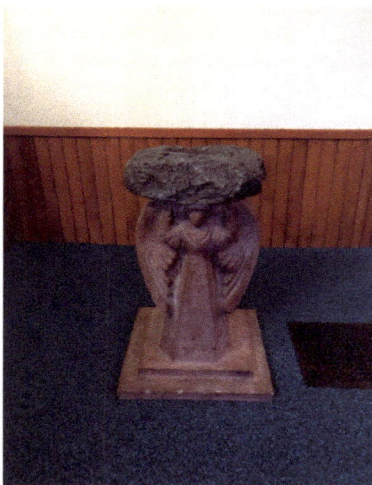

My thanks to Reverend Karen Fournier, minister of Oxford Congregational Church, for the photograph of the baptismal font.

The assistance of many friends, yet unmet, have made this work a pleasure.

Change helplessness to hopefulness.

Joslin was ahead of his time in organising and pioneering treatment of diabetes by a team including the patient, a nurse, dietician and chemist. The chemist is yet to make his mark in the treating team even today! Joslin placed the patient at the centre of the team.

A diabetic is his own nurse and chemist but if he tries to be the doctor he will come to grief.

Instructions to patients were clear and at times even blunt.

Help the doctor and you help yourself.

Emphasising education rather than providing instruction without explanation, Joslin practised and preached patience and compassion, especially when it came to young people.

Here he quotes from Solomon's soliloquy, Proverbs 16:32.

He that is slow to anger is better than the mighty; and he that ruleth his spirit than he that taketh a city.

Unlike most quotes and aphorisms which are found in the manuals, the following two are from Joslin's textbook, *The Treatment of Diabetes Mellitus,* perhaps to provide support for doctors when challenged.

Joslin's retort to "laugh and grow fat" was *"be thin, and laugh longer."*

Also, *"Decrease your waist-line to increase your life-line."*

In some of his writings Joslin listed a series of rules which he called the diabetic creed. These were more for the guidance of doctors. In the manuals he is much more specific, as he is in this aphorism.

Escape obesity by leaving the table a little early, avoiding second helpings and sodas.

Apollinaire Bouchardat (1809–1886) had advocated teaching patients with diabetes to manage their condition in the context of everyday needs. He treated disadvantaged patients at Hotel Dieu, a hospital established by a religious order in the seventh century and which remains in service to this day. Bouchardat worked to the end of his life. He died penniless.

Joslin called him "the prince of physicians," and visited his grave in the Pere Lachaise Cemetery whenever he visited Paris.

Here he is quoting the French physician's recommendation for exercise.

"One should exercise, preferably three times a day – in the forenoon , early afternoon, and evening – long enough to get warm but not tired ".

Joslin had attended Yale College (class of 1890). The curriculum included Latin and Greek. The aphorism here is the English translation of one of the sayings of Virgil. It refers to one consequence of falling into temptation which, in the case of patients with diabetes, most commonly referred to dietary indiscretions.

Descent into hell is easy.

This, according to those who worked with him, described Joslin's favourite activity.

Gladly would he learn and gladly teach.

Joslin was an admirer of Gandhi, the Indian politician and activist known for engaging in prolonged fasting as a form of dissent. Another way to express the same sentiment was to practise what one preached. Joslin was known for his self-restraint. His weight remained a steady 140 pounds for most of his adult life. He did not smoke, and abstained from alcohol.

"Be the change you want to see." MK Gandhi.

Motto used in the first edition of *Principles and Practice of Medicine,* the textbock for medical students written by Sir William Osler in 1892 and used by Joslin when he was a medical student.

And I said of medicine, that this is an art which considers the constitution of the patient, and has principles of action and reason in each case. Plato, Gorgias.

Joslin served in the US armed forces in the First World War from February 1918 to March 1919. He was discharged with the rank of Lieutenant-Colonel, MC, US Army.

Life on the front taught me that worry does not cause diabetes.

Joslin encouraged self-reliance and expected his patients to take charge of their diabetes.

In early 1927 an 11-year-old girl was referred to Joslin for treatment shortly after the onset of diabetes. She showed him a photograph of herself holding a pet lion cub. Joslin included that photograph in every one of his manuals over a period of 25 years. This comment was printed below the photograph.

If a diabetic child can control a lion she can certainly control diabetes.

In the manuals Joslin studiously avoided technical terms and never talked down to patients. He expressed admiration for Browning's language in the latter's "author's apology." Joslin said, "I only wish that my language was as simple and that I could say to my patients as he to his readers for nearly 300 years."

"Art thou forgetful? Wouldst thou remember
From New-year's-day to the last of December?
Then read my Fancies, they will stick like Burrs,
And may be to the Helpless, Comforters."

Today the cost of providing treatment for diabetes and its complications is a major challenge for most developed countries.

Joslin saw this more than 100 years ago.

In the first edition of his manual, published in 1918, he said that the number of patients in the United States was "not far from half a million".

Current (2020) estimates of diabetes in the United States place the number in excess of 30 million.

The danger of growing old, whether diabetic or non-diabetic, is now double what it was in 1860 and hence it is part of wisdom that all prepare for a long life.

Treatment of Diabetes Mellitus. E P Joslin, 1928

Joslin always knew the importance of laboratory research. He had come under the influence of the brilliant physiologist, R H Chittenden, at Yale. The value of laboratory work was reinforced by his visits to the European centres beginning in the year following graduation and continued throughout his professional life.

Progress in diabetes always begins in the laboratory.

Joslin set high standards for his staff and, some would say, also for his patients, but no higher than those he set for himself.

If I miss a vein when collecting blood from a patient I immediately give him three dollars.

He believed in hard work, as evidenced by the prodigious output of his writings at the same time as he developed his three- pronged practice of clinical care in the office and hospital, camps for diabetic children and a research facility.

The greatest insurance for happiness is hard work.

At his country estate, Buffalo Hill, Joslin ran a fully-fledged working farm where he had sheep, horses, cattle, pigs and poultry as well as crops. "Joslin is our leading poultry farmer," declared one of his neighbours in Oxford.

As noted by Donald M Barnett in *Elliott P. Joslin, MD: A Centennial Portrait,* Joslin was fond of using agrarian metaphors.

No farmer can fatten hogs without overfeeding them.

Joslin had a large network of friends and acquaintances, not only in the medical field but also in research and non-medical circles including government officials. He also kept closely in touch with colleagues in general (primary care) practice. A general practitioner, Dr Sabine, who practised in Brookline, a suburb near Joslin's office, told Joslin that among his patients those who favoured outdoor activities such as camping usually had better control of their diabetes.

When a man is promoted from an outdoor position to an office, he becomes a candidate for diabetes.

Although a lifelong teetctaller, in his final years Joslin, on one occasion, served sherry to his colleagues when they visited his home in Longwood Towers.

Total abstinence is easier to follow than having an occasional drink – as is a strict diet without "occasional breaks".

Convinced of the value of education of the patient as an effective method for treating diabetes, Joslin also pioneered the use of summer camps for diabetic children. In addition to lectures on practical aspects of managing diabetes with insulin and exercise, he also saw the camps as a way of lightening the burden of the parents of diabetic children during the summer months. Many other institutions quickly followed his example.

Both the girls' camp, named after Clara Barton, and the boys', named – at the insistence of the benefactors – after Joslin, remain fully operational to this day.

It will take a combination of many minds to extend the bounds of knowledge of diabetes by a discovery equal to that of insulin.

Early in his professional career Joslin was struck by the quiet acceptance of their condition by his younger patients.

Therefore, like children, face the facts, accept the situation, study the disease and become masters of your fate.

In 1920 a 79-year-old woman called Louisa Drumm came to see Joslin for treatment of her recently discovered diabetes. She was taught to test her urine for glucose and other basics of treatment. Many years later a young man came to Joslin for treatment and told him that he was one of the 10 boarders in the boarding house run by Drumm. He told him that she had tested all of them the day after she came back from Boston and he was the only one found to have diabetes. Joslin's comment?

"Can one not appropriately say to younger diabetic patients go thou and do likewise?"

Diabetes should be a community responsibility.

In his senior years Joslin was inclined to lapse into reflections. In the ninth edition of his manual, when he was 84, he quoted from *Ulysses,* a poem by Tennyson. It was after he recounted the story of Louisa Drumm (p.70).

"Tho much is taken, much abides; and tho'
We are not now that strength which in the old days
 Moved earth and heaven, that which we are, we are,-
…. Made weak by time and fate, but strong in will."

Even when close to 90 years old Joslin kept up with the latest in research and developments in the treatment of diabetes. In the 10th edition of his manual he mentioned the establishment by Professor Raoul Boulin of a new clinic in Paris devoted to preventing diabetes. The quote opposite is attributed to Boulin.

"Le medecin arrive trop tard."

One should cease saying "the doctor arrived too late."

The opening line of Joslin's first instruction manual for diabetic patients in 1918.

For one diabetic who knows too much about his disease there are unquestionably ninety-nine who know too little.

The opening line of Joslin's final manual for diabetic patients written 40 years later (1959).

"It is seldom a diabetic patient returns whom I have treated as well as I might, or one who has followed treatment as well as he could."

Joslin befriended Charles Best when the latter was a medical student and participated in the discovery of insulin. The friendship lasted throughout Joslin's life. Best, who kept in touch with the Joslin family even after Joslin's death, is quoted in many of the manuals as he is here.

"The action of insulin is to remove all signs and symptoms of diabetes."

A brilliant student, Joslin never lost sight of the importance of developing a capacity for working long hours. He usually started work before daybreak and seldom went to bed before midnight.

Brains count. But knowledge alone will not save the diabetic.

This is a disease which tests the character of the patient, and for success in withstanding it, in addition to wisdom, he must possess honesty, self-control and courage. These qualities are as essential along with insulin as without insulin. (Manual, sixth edition, 1937 p. 14)

Joslin's meticulous records were used by a leading life insurance company to estimate the lifespan of diabetics. Joslin's comment on his mother's attitude to treatment and the effect of careful control on life expectancy is contained in his quote.

"I never knew her to break (her diet)…… She lived healthfully and cheerfully for 13 years with her diabetes which was as long as she was expected to live without it."

Repeatedly Joslin emphasised the importance of avoiding breaking the basic rules of treatment of diabetes by strict adherence to the prescribed program as seen in the next two aphorisms.

There is nothing which effort and unceasing and diligent care cannot overcome. (Seneca)

Another aphorism from the writings of Louis Pasteur.

These three things, Will, Work, Success, fill human existence.

He repeatedly emphasised the three basic tenets of treatment of diabetes, namely exercise, insulin and diet.

This quote was contained in a letter to Joslin by one of his patients.

"It is very hard to start the exercise, and the less one feels inclined to start it the more one needs it."

The simplicity of Joslin's instructions for patients was exemplary.

Sugar enters blood as fast as a child runs.

Starch (in bread) enters blood as fast as a child walks.

Starch in vegetables enters blood as fast as a child creeps.

To emphasise the importance of never neglecting the care of their diabetes Joslin quoted the philosopher William James (1842–1910).

"Every smallest stroke of virtue or vice leaves its ever so little scar... Nothing we ever do is in strict scientific literalness, wiped out."

Joslin encouraged young doctors to avoid restricting themselves to specialities in the early years of training. Here he provides his reason for saying so.

"To be a good specialist, a doctor first has to be a good general practitioner.

Diabetics like most people have all kinds of troubles and so when faced by a problem of which the diabetic complains, I take for granted that diabetes is not the whole story."

Even before specialising in diabetes Joslin had recognised an important difference between diabetes in children and diabetes in middle age, as can be seen in the next two quotes.

Unlike children, diabetics in middle life are proverbially fat before the disease begins.

In Joslin's time testing for sugar in the urine required the patient or his parents to know the method of using chemicals to make the determination. Tablets, then strips for that purpose came later. As for checking blood glucose, blood had to be sent to a laboratory.

It is a common occurrence for sugar to appear in the urine when a patient is gaining weight.

Joslin continued to emphasise the importance of treating even mild diabetes, convinced that it was going to slow down or even reverse the condition. This remains unappreciated even today.

Combat the slightest hint of diabetes.

As noted earlier, Joslin was one of the first physicians to document the rise in the incidence of diabetes. The following quote is from Don Barnett's *Elliott P. Joslin, MD: A Centennial Portrait.*

"Although six of seven persons, all head of families succumbed to diabetes, no one spoke of an epidemic...Consider the measures which would have been adopted to discover the source of the outbreak to prevent a recurrence.....if these deaths had occurred from scarlet fever, typhoid or tuberculosis....Because the disease was diabetes, and because the deaths occurred over a considerable interval of time, the fatalities passed unnoticed."

E P Joslin,1921

Repeatedly he urged that diabetic children be treated with compassion, even leniency, when it came to less than ideal adherence to the prescribed restrictions. He said, "Diabetic children mean to be honest. Children eventually will tell whether they have done right or wrong, but don't force them to do so."

"Do not rejoice when your enemy falls,

And let not your heart be glad when he stumbles…"

Proverbs 24:17

Joslin was always conscious of the importance of research and confident of continuing improvement in the understanding and treatment of diabetes.

No one expects that diabetes will be treated 10 years from now as it is today.

Even after seeing several hundred thousand diabetics over a lifetime of medical practice Joslin remained humble.

Transgression of the diet is frequently the fault of the doctor ("and of course I am here referring to myself"), for not explaining it clearly enough.

Looking over his career, one can clearly see that as time went on Joslin spent more and more time thinking about the best way to manage diabetes in children.

Every child has three mischievous ponies to drive and their names are diet, exercise and insulin (just as are the diabetic horses of the adult diabetic.) To harmonise the capriciousness of three such ponies is a tremendous triumph.

In spite of following a strict routine in his personal habits as well as in the care of his patients, Joslin was always open to the possibility of new ideas – even out of left field!

Here he quotes President A. Lawrence Lowell of Harvard University on "how knowledge progresses unwittingly…" in the ninth edition of his manual (p.87).

"... As has been said of Columbus, that when he started on his voyage he did not know where he was going, when he got there he did not know where he was, and when he got back he did not know where he had been; and yet he discovered America. Like his, the action was intentional, and in its direct objects perfectly logical, but led naturally to results wholly unexpected..."

According to the late Michael Bliss, who wrote *Harvey Cushing A Life in Surgery,* Cushing was a lifelong admirer of Joslin. Both had been part of a fundraising committee for student accommodation. Joslin attributed this aphorism to "my friend Dr Harvey Cushing".

Do not ask for a donation before the prospective donor has eaten. The heart is closer to the stomach than to the brain.

H G Wells, the well-known English novelist who suffered from diabetes, said human history is "a race between education and catastrophe."

Diabetic education for the patient and his carers was probably Joslin's greatest contribution to the management of diabetes.

"With a missionary zeal, one must convert not only the patient's mind and soul, but also his doctor to the realisation that it is worth the effort to control the disease as shown by the sugar-free urine, normal blood sugar and cholesterol."

Elliott P Joslin, 1959

"Elliott Proctor Joslin, pioneer medical specialist in diabetes mellitus died in his sleep on January 29, 1962 at his Longwood Towers home".

DM Barnett (From *Elliott P. Joslin, MD:A Centennial Portrait*.)

It is fitting that this collection of Joslin's sayings should end with a quote from Dr Donald M Barnett. Don came out of retirement to help preserve and curate Joslin's papers and other memorabilia which are preserved in the Joslin archives in the Marble Library at the Joslin Diabetes Centre in Boston. Sadly, ill health has prevented Don from completing his work on Joslin's remarkable life. Without his generous help and encouragement my attempts to present the Joslin story in *Joslin A Pioneer in Diabetes Care* (2019), would have been impossible.

Acknowledgement

Once again I gratefully acknowledge the kindness and generosity of the Joslin Diabetes Centre in permitting me access to the material in the archives. The Joslin archivist Matthew Brown was tireless in his efforts to provide documents, books and photographs at the time of my visit in 2014 and also after I returned to Sydney.

Shailendra K Sinha
Sydney, Australia
2020